As you begin to pay attention to your own

stories and what they say about you, you

will enter into the exciting process of becoming,

as you should be, the author of your own

life, the creator of your own possibilities.

MANDY AFTEL

ACKNOWLEDGEMENTS
These quotations were gathered lovingly but unscientifically
over several years and/or were contributed by many friends or
acquaintances. Some arrived—and survived in our files—on scraps
of paper and may therefore be imperfectly worded or attributed.
To the authors, contributors and original sources, our thanks and,
where appropriate, our apologies. —The Editors

WITH SPECIAL THANKS TO THE ENTIRE COMPENDIUM FAMILY.

CREDITS

Compiled by: Dan Zadra

Designed by: Steve Potter

ISBN: 978-1-932319-68-2

2nd Printing. Printed in China with soy inks.

HOPE every day.

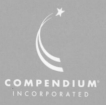

Hope is
the voice of
the heart.

You are alive,
and that is
the only place
you need to be
to start.

CARRIE RAINEY

HOPE every day.

The moment
you survive the
diagnosis you
become a
survivor. The
moment your
cancer has
been detected,
your success
story begins.

VICKIE GIRARD

HOPE every day.

Hope is a
reaffirmation
of life.

KELLY ANN ROTHAUS

HOPE every day.

The capacity for
hope is the most
significant fact
of life. It provides
human beings
with a sense of
destination and
the energy to
get started.

NORMAN COUSINS

HOPE every day.

Faith is the
very first thing
you should pack
in a hope chest.

SARAH BAN BREATHNACH

To succeed,
we must first
believe that
we can.

MICHAEL KORDA

HOPE every day.

Believe there's
light at the
end of the
tunnel. Believe
that you might
be that light for
someone else.

KOBI YAMADA

HOPE every day.

If there is hope
in the future,
there is power
in the present.

JOHN MAXWELL

HOPE every day.

Embrace the
sorrow for
awhile and
then let go
and get to
work on it.

PAT COVINA

HOPE every day.

We shall
draw from the
heart of suffering
itself the means
of inspiration
and survival.

WINSTON CHURCHILL

HOPE every day.

Life's challenges
are not supposed
to paralyze us,
they're supposed
to help us discover
who we are.

BERNICE JOHNSON REAGON

HOPE every day.

Things don't
go wrong so
you can give up.
They happen to
break you down
and build you
up so you can
be all that you
were intended
to be.

CHARLES JONES

HOPE every day.

What I have
now, I know
that no army
can take from
me. I have
myself.

MICHAEL J. FOX

HOPE every day.

Within you
lies a power
greater than
what lies
before you.

RHONDA BLAKE

HOPE every day.

Hope begins in
the dark...if you
just show up and
try to do the right
thing, the dawn
will come. You
wait and watch
and work; you
don't give up.

ANNE LAMOTT

HOPE every day.

So if there is
a purpose to
the suffering that
is cancer, I think
it must be this:
it's meant to
improve us.

LANCE ARMSTRONG

HOPE every day.

Cancer is not a
death sentence,
but rather it is
a life sentence;
it pushes one
to live.

MARCIA SMITH

HOPE every day.

My cancer scare
changed my life.
I'm grateful for
every new, healthy
day I have. It
has helped me
prioritize my life.

OLIVIA NEWTON-JOHN

HOPE every day.

By fighting cancer
you are moving
one of life's bad
events into the
past column and
getting ready for
some of the good.

VICKIE GIRARD

HOPE every day.

God did not
make us to be
eaten up by
anxiety, but to
walk, unafraid
in a world where
there is work to
do, and love to
give and win.

JOSEPH FORT NEWTON

HOPE every day.

Once you
choose hope,
anything's
possible.

CHRISTOPHER REEVE

HOPE every day.

We are
living with—
not dying of—
cancer.

Hope ever
urges us on
and tells us
tomorrow will
be better.

TIBULLUS

HOPE every day.

For I know
the plans I
have for you;
plans to prosper
you and not to
harm you,
plans to give
you hope and
a future.

JEREMIAH 29:11

HOPE every day.

Compassion for
myself is the
most powerful
healer of them all.

THEODORE ISAAC RUBIN

HOPE every day.

I need to take an
emotional breath,
step back, and
remind myself
who's actually in
charge of my life.

JUDITH M. KNOWLTON

HOPE every day.

How do we
nurture the soul?
By revering our
own life. By
learning to live
it all, not only
the joys and the
victories, but also
the pain and the
struggle.

NATHANIEL BRANDEN, PH.D.

HOPE every day.

Know that
you yourself
are a miracle.

NORMAN VINCENT PEALE

HOPE every day.

Trust in your own
untried capacity.

ELLA WHEELER WILCOX

HOPE every day.

You got
yourself this
far—you just
got to keep
going.

DON WARD

HOPE every day.

I don't look
at what I've
lost. I look
instead at what
I have left.

BETTY FORD

HOPE every day.

So much of our
journey is the
hard work of
learning about
and removing
barriers.

MELODY BEATTIE

HOPE every day.

Hope can
always cope.

P.K. THOMAJAN

HOPE every day.

I was always
looking outside
myself for
strength and
confidence
but it comes
from within.
It is there all
the time.

ANNA FREUD

HOPE every day.

There is much
in the world to
make us afraid.
There is much
more in our faith
to make us unafraid.

FREDERICK W. CROPP

HOPE every day.

Real difficulties
can be overcome,
it is only the
imaginary
ones that are
unconquerable.

THEODORE N. VAIL

HOPE every day.

I have learned
to live each day
as it comes,
and not to
borrow trouble
by dreading
tomorrow.

DOROTHY DIX

HOPE every day.

Every evening I
turn my worries
over to God.
He's going to
be up all night
anyway.

MARY CROWLEY

HOPE every day.

When you have
done your best,
await the result
in peace.

FRANK VIZZARE

HOPE every day.

How simple
it is to see
that we can
only be happy
now, and that
there will never
be a time when
it is not now.

GERALD JAMPOLSKY

HOPE every day.

Laughter
is part of
the human
survival kit.

DAVID NATHAN

HOPE every day.

I have seen
what a laugh
can do. It can
transform almost
unbearable tears
into something
bearable, even
hopeful.

BOB HOPE

HOPE every day.

As humans,
we sometimes
stand tall and
look into the
sun and laugh,
and I think we
are never more
brave than when
we do that.

LINDA ELLERBEE

HOPE every day.

There are really
only two ways to
approach life—
as a victim or as a
gallant fighter...

MERLE SHAIN

HOPE every day.

Everyday courage
has few witnesses.
But yours is no
less noble because
no drum beats
before you, and
no crowds shout
your name.

ROBERT LOUIS STEVENSON

HOPE every day.

The more serious
the illness, the
more important
it is for you to
fight back, mobilizing
all your resources—
spiritual, emotional,
intellectual, physical.

NORMAN COUSINS

HOPE every day.

Hope is not
a feeling,
it's something
you do.

KATHERINE PATERSON

HOPE every day.

God, give me guts.

ELI MYGATT

HOPE every day.

Toughness is
in the soul
and spirit, not
in muscles.

ALEX KARRAS

HOPE every day.

A strong
positive mental
attitude will
create more
miracles than
any wonder
drug.

PATRICIA NEAL

HOPE every day.

Optimism is
the foundation
of courage.

NICHOLAS MURRAY BUTLER

HOPE every day.

I now know
that we can
train our
thoughts to be
our biggest
allies and work
for us, not
against us.

VICKIE GIRARD

HOPE every day.

Never talk
defeat.
Use words
like hope,
belief, faith,
victory.

NORMAN VINCENT PEALE

HOPE every day.

We may have
cancer, but
cancer does
not have us.

RALLY SIGN

HOPE every day.

Give us grace
and strength to
forbear and to
persevere...give
us courage...and
the quiet mind.

ROBERT LOUIS STEVENSON

HOPE every day.

I am very
aware that we
can only think
one thought
at a time. So I
refuse to think
the negative
thoughts that
keep the good
out.

LOUISE L. HAY

HOPE every day.

Sometimes our
light goes out
but is blown into
flame by another
human being. Each
of us owes deepest
thanks to those
who have rekindled
this inner light.

ALBERT SCHWEITZER

HOPE every day.

Treasure the one
who believed in
you when you
ceased to believe
in yourself.

UNKNOWN

HOPE every day.

Friendship gives
value to survival.

C.S. LEWIS

HOPE every day.

Trouble is a
part of your
life, and if you
don't share
it, you don't
give the person
who loves you
enough chance
to love you
enough.

DINAH SHORE

HOPE every day.

Hope can
open the door
to change, so
surround yourself
with people
who share your
hopes. Love can
do anything, so
surround yourself
with people who
love and care
for you.

DAN ZADRA

HOPE every day.

Fear is useless.
Faith is necessary.
Love is everything.

MARTIN SHEEN

HOPE every day.

You are loved.
If so, what
else matters?

UNKNOWN

The feeling
remains that
God is on the
journey, too.

ST. TERESA OF AVILA

HOPE every day.

Faith is not a
pill you take,
but a muscle
you use.

UNKNOWN

HOPE every day.

I believe in
the sun even
if it isn't shining.
I believe in love
even when I am
alone. I believe
in God even when
He is silent.

WORLD WAR II REFUGEE

HOPE every day.

God has faith
in you. He
proved it by
giving you life.

PETE ZAFRA

HOPE every day.

It gets dark
sometimes, but
morning comes.
Don't you surrender!
Keep hope alive.

JESSE JACKSON

HOPE every day.

In the darkest
hour the soul is
replenished and
given the strength
to continue and
endure.

HEART WARRIOR CHOSA

HOPE every day.

If you're going
through hell,
keep on going.

RODNEY ATKINS

HOPE every day.

I will persist.
I will always
take another step.
If that is of no
avail I will take
another, and
yet another.

OG MANDINO

HOPE every day.

Life begins on
the other side
of despair.

JEAN-PAUL SARTRE

HOPE every day.

Hope is the
feeling you have
that the feeling
you have isn't
permanent.

JEAN KERR

HOPE every day.

Hope returns
with the sun.

JUVENAL

HOPE every day.

Every day holds
the possibility
of a miracle.

ELIZABETH DAVID

HOPE every day.

Each dawn
holds a new
hope for a new
plan, making
the start of each
day the start of
a new life.

GINA BLAIR

HOPE every day.

Count not
what is lost but
what is left.

THEODORE LAU

HOPE every day.

Light tomorrow
with today.

ELIZABETH BARRETT BROWNING

HOPE every day.

Every day is
a leap of faith.

LIZZ WRIGHT

HOPE every day.

Some days there
won't be a song
in your heart.
Sing anyway.

EMORY AUSTIN

HOPE every day.

Even if
happiness
forgets you a
little bit, never
completely
forget about it.

JACQUES PRÉVERT

Every day that we
wake up is a good
day. Every breath
that we take is
filled with hope
for a better day.

WALTER MOSLEY

HOPE every day.

Either you
reach a higher
point today, or
you exercise
your strength in
order to be able
to climb higher
tomorrow.

FRIEDRICH NIETZSCHE

Some things
have to be
believed to
be seen.

RALPH HODGSON

HOPE every day.

Faith sees
the invisible,
believes the
incredible, and
receives the
impossible.

MARTIN LUTHER

I urge you to
be challenged
and inspired
by what you do
not know.

MICHAEL J. FOX

HOPE every day.

All I have seen
teaches me to
trust the Creator
for all I have
not seen.

RALPH WALDO EMERSON

HOPE every day.

Never let the
word "impossible"
stop you from
pursuing what
your heart and
spirit urge you
to do. Impossible
things come true
every day.

ROBERT K. COOPER

HOPE every day.

It is difficult
to say what is
impossible, for
the dream of
yesterday is the
hope of today
and the reality
of tomorrow.

ROBERT H. GODDARD

We are never helpless.

DR. TOM G. STEVENS

HOPE every day.

There are
no hopeless
situations;
there are only
people who have
grown hopeless
about them.

CLARE BOOTHE LUCE

HOPE every day.

I discovered
I always have
choices and
sometimes it's
only a choice
of attitude.

JUDITH M. KNOWLTON

HOPE every day.

If you can't
make it better,
you can laugh at
it. And if you can
laugh at it, you
can live with it.

ERMA BOMBECK

HOPE every day.

You may have to
fight a battle more
than once to win it.

MARGARET THATCHER

HOPE every day.

Nobody is stronger
than someone
who came back...
nothing can be
done to such a
person because
whatever you could
do is less than
what has already
been done.

ELIE WIESEL

HOPE every day.

There is nothing
more beautiful in
life than getting a
second chance.

RON KOVIC

HOPE every day.

Persistence is
the hard work
you do after
you've finished
doing the hard
work you did.

FAITH BAILEY

HOPE every day.

The greatest
things ever done
on earth have been
done little by little.

THOMAS GUTHRIE

HOPE every day.

Victory is won
not in miles but in
inches. Win a little
now, hold your
ground, and later
win a little more.

LOUIS L'AMOUR

HOPE every day.

Remember that
what is hard to
endure will be
sweet to recall.

UNKNOWN

One day,
in retrospect
the years of
struggle will
strike you as the
most beautiful.

SIGMUND FREUD

HOPE every day.

Look back,
and smile on
perils past.

SIR WALTER SCOTT

Things will
usually come
out all right,
but sometimes
it takes strong
nerves just to
watch.

HEDLEY DONOVAN

Tears may be
dried up, but the
heart—never.

MARGUERITE DE VALOIS

HOPE every day.

When I stand
before you at the
day's end, you
shall see my scars
and know that I
had my wounds
and also my healing.

RABINDRANATH TAGORE

HOPE every day.

As cancer
patients we
are different,
now. These
circumstances
have changed
us, that is true.
But we aren't
anything less,
we are more.

VICKIE GIRARD

HOPE every day.

May you live
all the days of
your life!

JONATHAN SWIFT

HOPE every day.

I am not afraid
of tomorrow, for I
have seen yesterday
and I love today.

WILLIAM ALLEN WHITE

HOPE every day.

The strongest and
sweetest songs yet
remain to be sung.

WALT WHITMAN

HOPE every day.